Learning more about Autism

Dealing with Autism in the Family

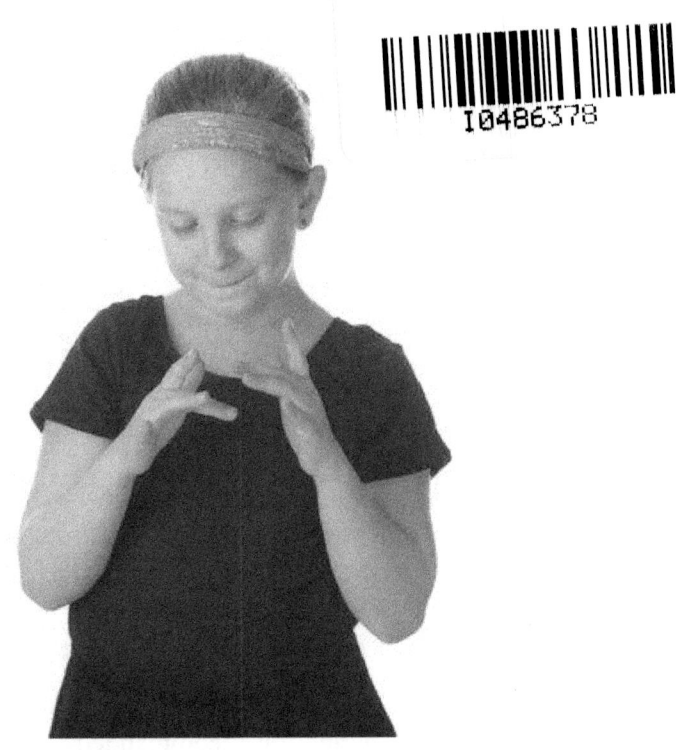

Healthy Learning Series

Dueep Jyot Singh

Mendon Cottage Books

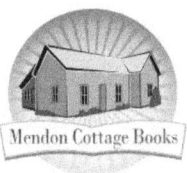

JD-Biz Publishing

Disclaimer

The information is this book is provided for informational purposes only. It is not intended to be used and medical advice or a substitute for proper medical treatment by a qualified health care provider. The information is believed to be accurate as presented based on research by the author.

The contents have not been evaluated by the U.S. Food and Drug Administration or any other Government or Health Organization and the contents in this book are not to be used to treat cure or prevent disease.

The author or publisher is not responsible for the use or safety of any diet, procedure or treatment mentioned in this book. The author or publisher is not responsible for errors or omissions that may exist.

Warning

The Book is for informational purposes only and before taking on any diet, treatment or medical procedure, it is recommended to consult with your primary health care provider.

Our books are available at

1. Amazon.com

2. Barnes and Noble

3. Itunes

4. Kobo

5. Smashwords

6. Google Play Books

Table of Contents

Introduction

Autism is a many times inherited disorder which becomes apparent in early childhood. Children suffering from autism are going to have a lot of problems in communicating verbally. This is a neuro- development disorder which is going to prevent children from learning and communicating in a verbal language, as well as understanding abstract concepts.

This book is going to give you more information about this disorder, its reasons, it symptoms, and how you can cope with a child suffering from autism in your family.

Definition of Autism

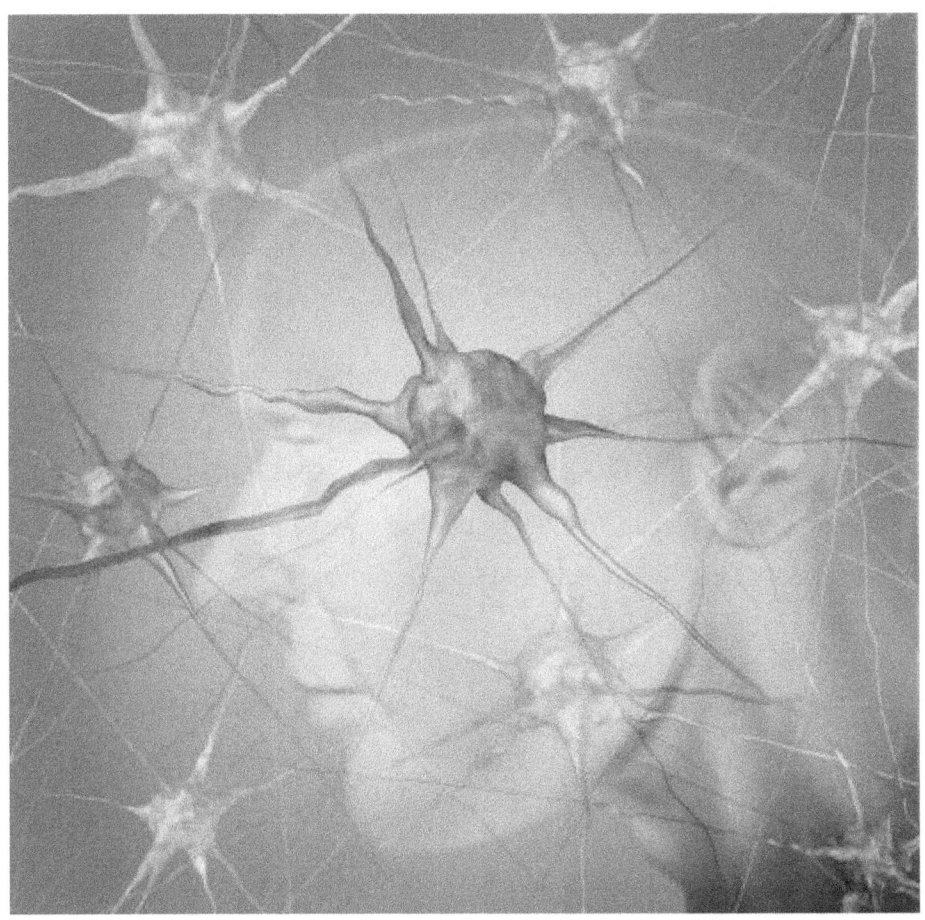

Autism is now known as Autism Spectrum Disorder [ASD]. It is a complex neurodevelopment disorder which is going to appear in a child during the first three years of his life.

This affects the development of that portion of your brain, which deals with social reciprocity and communication skills. This is one of the five disorders that constitute Pervasive Development Disorders [PDD.] The other four disorders are Asperger's Disorder, Childhood Disintegrative Disorder [CDD], Rett's Disorder and PDD- Not Otherwise Specified (PDD-NOS), as defined by the Autism Society of America.

The severity can range from mild, moderate to severe. Roughly 70% of these children are going to have an intelligence level, which normal people consider to fall in the mental retardation range. That is because their mental development has been interrupted somewhere and it causes the interference of the development of language, which may be slow or abnormal.

Jennifer's 14-year-old son was diagnosed with autism when he was 1 ½ years old. According to her, he was tested when he was a baby, because he had not begun speaking words by the age of 12 – 18 months. A child specialist, told his parents that his feeble voice was due to possible non-development of his vocal cords, and suggested that he get checked up by a specialist for possible autism.

After the diagnosis of autism is confirmed in her son, Jennifer went through training to teach her child with special needs and now she trains others children suffering from autism.

She says that many of these children are excellent in some skills. They are intelligent; they may like one particular subject and language. They may be geniuses in creative arts. The only problem is that they are going to be nonverbal and that is why many times, specialists suggest the using of pictorial cards to help them communicate and indicate what they want.

The only problem is because autism also has its side effects of impaired nonverbal, verbal communication, and social interaction, repetitive and often restricted behavior, many people in ignorance consider this to be a form of mental sickness.

In medieval times, the child suffering from autism would have been killed because he/she was possessed by the devil. That was because his/her attempts to communicate and wanting to tell you about his/her needs, along with jerky movements would be read as the possession of the devil, who had taken over the body and soul of an innocent child.

It is said that a priest spoke with a child who had been possessed by the devil because he lived in a fantasy world of his own. He was considered to be "a soulless lump of flesh" because he could not speak properly. He advocated this child be killed. Some people consider this story to be apocryphal, but even if it was half true, one can only understand about how a child with developmental problems in the medieval ages would fare in that ignorant and devil ridden social atmosphere.

Luckily, we are in the 21st century, and parents are more conscious and knowledgeable about this disorder today. That is why sensible parents are always on the lookout for supposedly "abnormal" behavior during the first 12 months of first child's existence. The symptoms are going to develop gradually. However, in many cases, some autistic children develop at the normal pace expected for a normal child, and after that, there is a regression.

They are not mentally retarded. They are not morons. I remember a woman who shied away from an autistic child by saying that she had a disgust of the mentally retarded. When she started to talk to me, I shied away from her saying that I was not in the habit of speaking with mentally challenged morons. I really did not have the time and the patience nor did I have the inclination to do so.

Who, me, she hooted in a very offended and *How Dare You Insult Me* manner. I told her that if she was ignorant enough not to know the difference between autism and the really mentally retarded, I could not credit her with great intellectual power. And I did not suffer fools gladly.

She is still not talking to me, because I affronted and slighted her so mortally. But this unfortunately is the general concept of people who are confronted with an autistic child for the first time. They immediately say in a very rude manner, "What is wrong with him? Is he mad or something? Why does he keep piling up blocks in a line? Why is he ignoring me? "

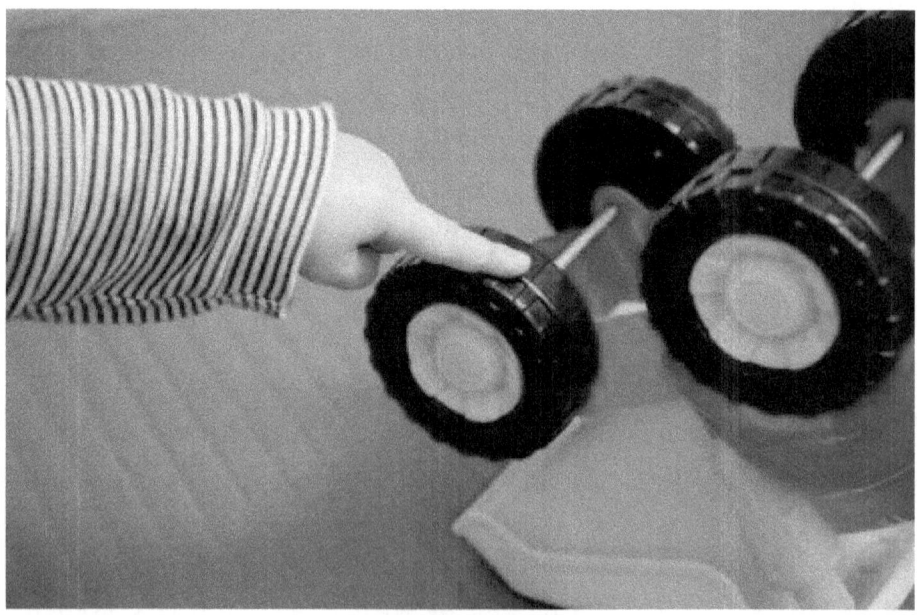

They do not know that this sort of repetitive behavior is one of the symptoms of autism. Children with autism are generally oblivious to their environment. They are definitely unaware of others feelings towards them.

Autistic children are poor academically, but they find it easier to communicate, musically. They are going to find it difficult to learn letters and they are not going to grasp any abstract concept. However, if you train them in creative skills, they are going to show a marked success in doing that particular activity, they like drawing, painting, doing embroidery, and singing.

Just as it takes all kinds of people to make the world, no two autistic people are going to display similar behavior abnormalities and skills. Though physically they may grow up, mentally they may be on the level of a normal child of 7 – 10.

Probable Causes of Autism

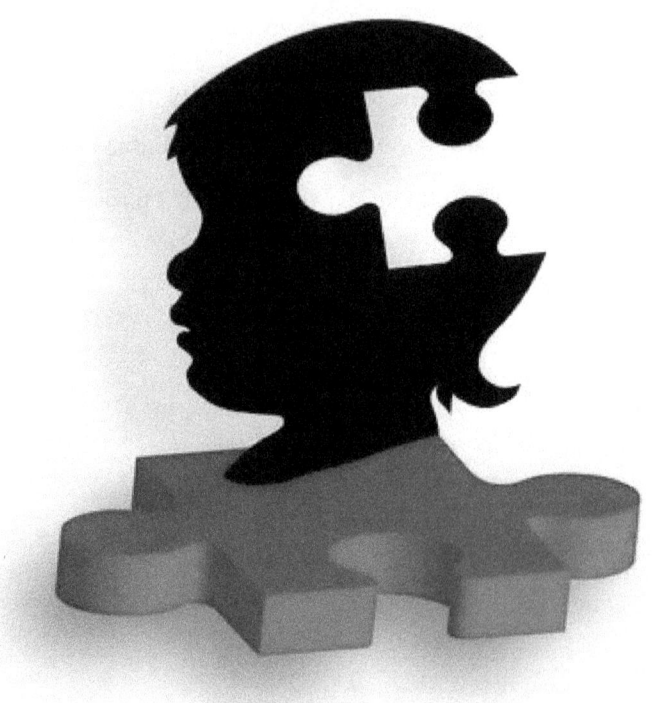

Autism is definitely not restricted to just one particular race or bloodline. However, it is considered to be inherited genetically, and 2 – 10 people out of every 10,000 people are going to suffer from some sort of autism, depending on the diagnostic criteria used., 4 times as many males as females are affected by this disorder – no matter the social or racial or genetic backgrounds.

Researchers suspect that apart from genetic factors, environmental circumstances are capable of autism in a child. In very rare cases, these defects are caused in a baby due to some external or internal agents like infection in the mother during gestation.

Vaccines definitely do not have anything to do with autism. Some years ago, a controversy stated that autism was related to vaccines, and many people earned plenty of compensation through malpractice suits. This was definitely a scam.

Also there is a rumor going around that some drugs and medicines taken by the mother during pregnancy cause autism in her child. After the thalidomide scare and terrible side effects of this drug, anybody can say anything about drugs affecting the mother and her unborn child. But there are some factors, which are going to alter the information processing system in the brain, especially if the child is genetically prone to autism.

Genetic Background

What doctors do know is that some children are vulnerable and parents can start getting signs of their delayed development very early. There are some genes being identified by autism by researchers. In one particular group of autism, children definitely have genetic origins of this disorder.

However, if you take the family history of a child with autism and look into the problem with his/her mother, father, grandparents, uncles, and aunts and ask for clear autism symptoms, there is a chance you may not get them!

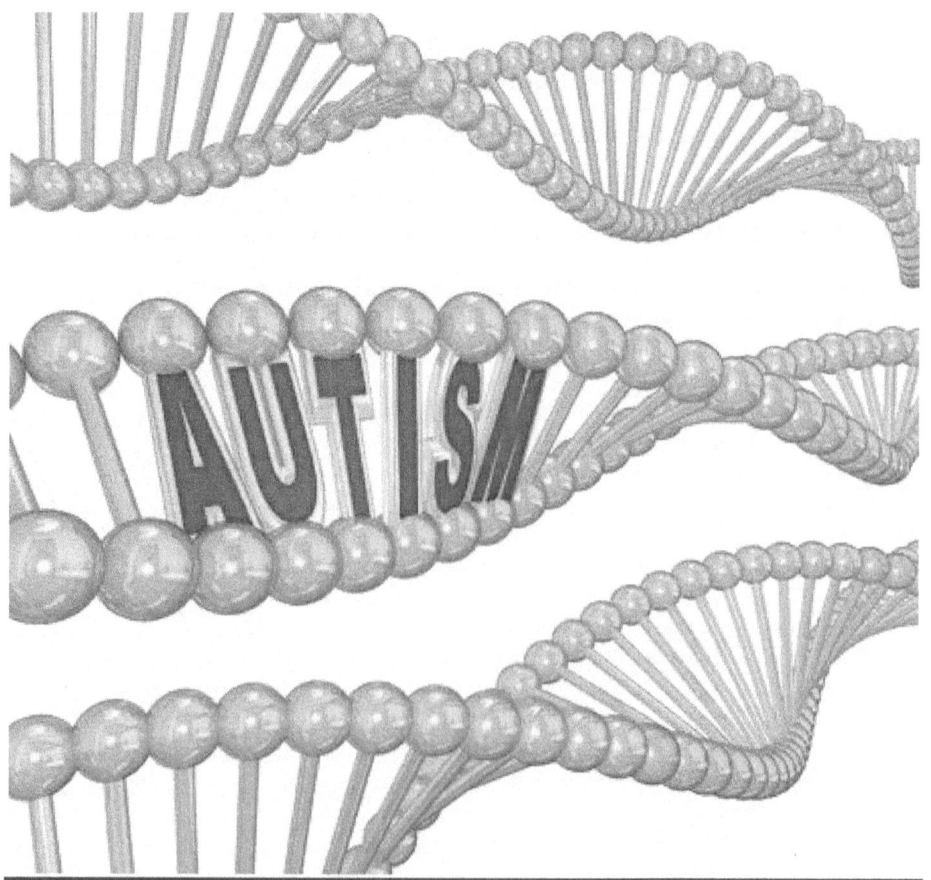

Many of these children born of autistic genes are normal. However, some of their siblings may show signs of autism. They are going to display some problems in socializing and communication. If the child starts showing these problems, it is better to look at your family members and ask whether there were some of them who had delayed speech or were considered to be odd or eccentric.

There must have been some relative who was supposedly highly shy. On the other hand, you may have this child showing symptoms totally different from any other behavioral disorders shown by members of the family in an autistic – prone bloodline.

All these individuals may not fall under the clear autism syndrome, but they may be what you call the broad form. This means that in some families where you have a child with autism, you are going to find a greater concentration of some of these deficits in the family members.

Apart from heredity, there are other factors which are being associated in the creation of conditions which affect brain development, occurring before, during or soon after birth. Some of these children may have biochemical and neurological abnormalities.

Symptoms of Autism

One in 68 children have been diagnosed to be suffering from autism in 2014, in the USA. This is a 30% higher rate than the children suffering in 2012, which was *One in 88*. This is getting to be a worrisome trend. It is disturbing to hear that the number of people who are being diagnosed with autism has increased dramatically, but whether they really do suffer from autism is a matter of conjecture, because ever since the government decided to subsidize financial bonuses and incentives for those children suffering from autism in the 1980s, the statistics have gone up!

This is not just my cynical sense talking. One still does not know how many people really suffer from this disorder.

People who are suffering from autism are not going to be disabled, physically. They look like anybody without the disability. There is no remission for this disorder even though they have been instances of people supposedly cured by doctors and trainers, but that is a statement, taken by a pinch of salt, by researchers and scientists.

An autistic child is going to be impaired severely in one particular field, but he is going to be superior or normal in other fields. That is why these children are called savants or "those who know" from the French verb savoir, which literally means "to know.""

The child is not going to respond to his name and often avoids making eye contact with people. But that does not mean that he does not wish to talk to you at that particular moment. It is just that his mind has not managed to give his eyes the "normal" social order to respond to a verbal command.

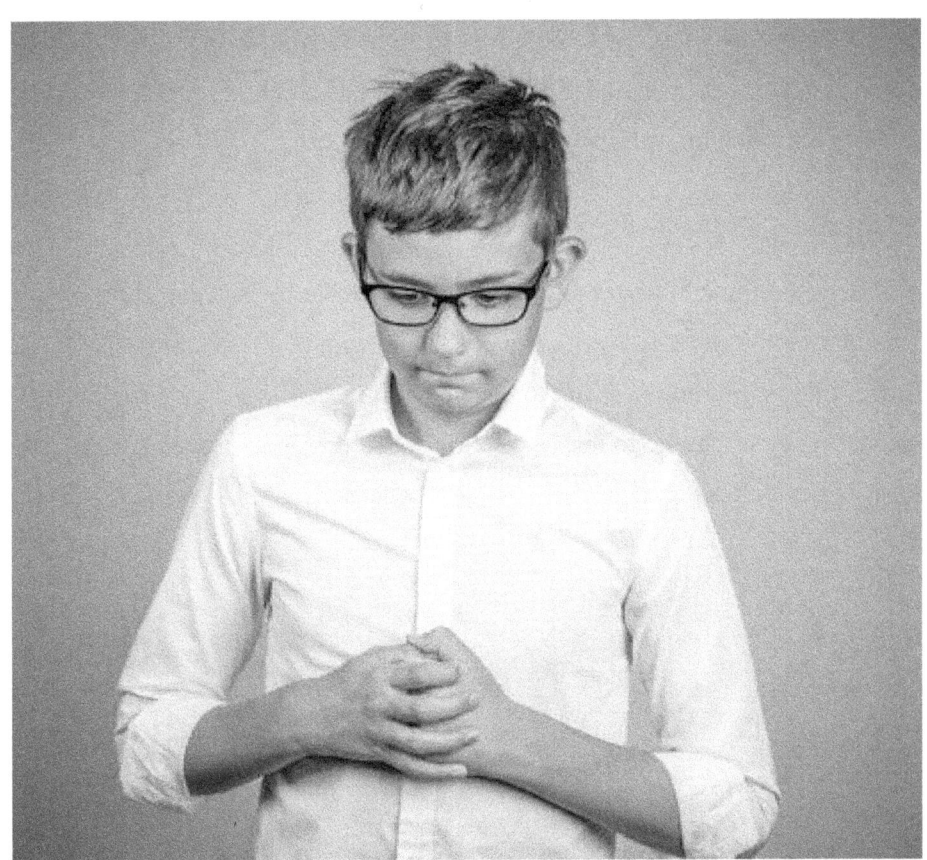

These children have restricted interests, and they often do certain actions repeatedly. For instance, they may keep fiddling with a pen or doing one particular action continuously and in a repetitive fashion.

The symptoms are going to show up by the time the baby is six months old. He is not going to respond when you call him. He is not going to speak or make any childlike noises. Some people even think that their autistic babies are deaf. That is not true. That is why any child being shouted at and not responding can possibly be autistic. Parents need to know this.

These symptoms are going to continue through babyhood and are going to develop in some form or the other, throughout adulthood, though it is going to be in a much more mild and muted form or shape.

Symptom Triad

The basic symptom Triad is an impairment of social interaction, communication skills, and repetitive behavior with restricted interests. A few of these children are going to have a great fascination for one article or subject. They are going to display a really good depth of knowledge about that subject of their choice.

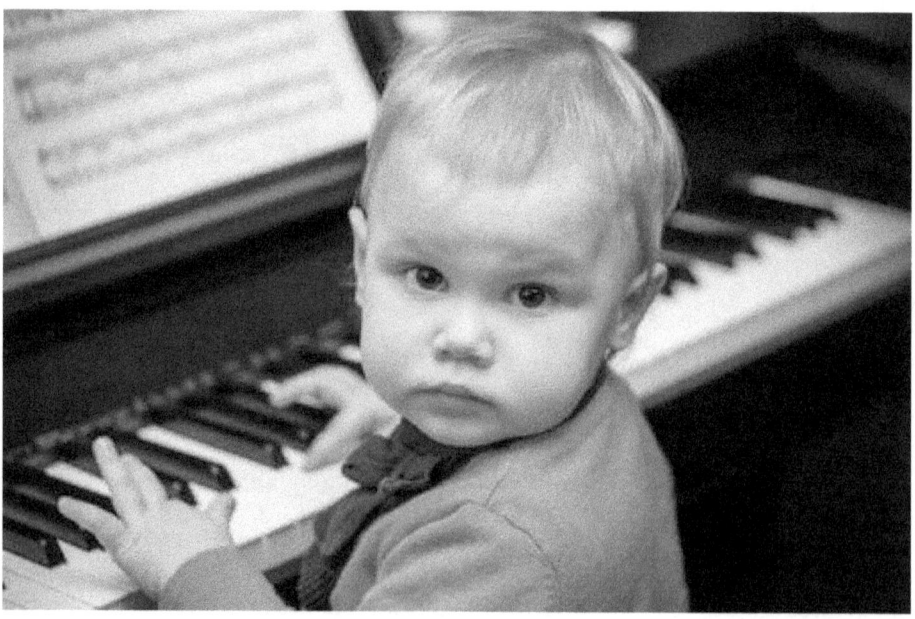

Some of these children have fantastic abilities, especially in the field of math, music, and memorizing things. A lot of autistic children love music.

Those who are verbal can learn a number of compositions, though the learning material may not have any communicative value.

They are going to know a lot about it, but they are not going to know much about other things they need to know or are supposed to know for their age and level group.

I know a six-year-old autistic child who lives, breathes and dreams of cats. She is fascinated with them. She communicates to us with meows, which are repetitive. Her drawings of cats is far superior than an average six-year-old child's rendition of cats' sketch work. Her concentration while drawing these cats is very good, and she could not care less about the world around her. However she is not going to tolerate any moving away of her meticulously lined up pens, sketch pens, paints, and papers.

Any such action is going to bring about crying, while she definitely does not look up to see your face.

Voice and Facial Response

Children with autism are not able to interpret the tone of your voice. They also do not understand facial expressions or your emotions. As they do not look directly at your face you cannot teach them cues about appropriate behavior.

Remember that this social development which one takes for granted in a normal child is not possible in an autistic child, because he/she is not mentally equipped in that particular area to recognize it.

So if your baby does not look at you when you call him/her, does not respond to your touch or any other social stimuli and smile like a normal child would do, look at their movements.

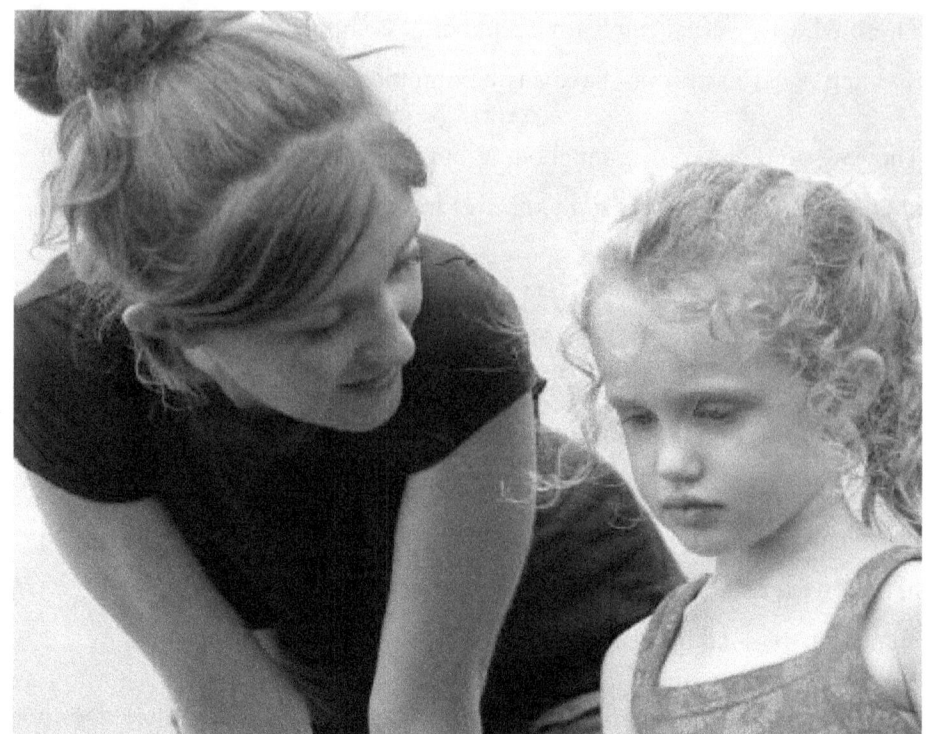

Do they point to things? A normal child is going to do that when he /she wants it. An autistic child cannot do that. Is their behavior repetitive? You may find these children lining up their toys in the same pattern again and again.

Children between the age group of 3 to 5 are not going to approach you spontaneously. They are not going to respond to your interactions with them, or to emotions. They are not going to imitate you. Their communication method is normally going to be nonverbal.

However, they are very affectionate, and they are going to be very deeply attached to the people who give them care, even though they cannot show it emotionally.

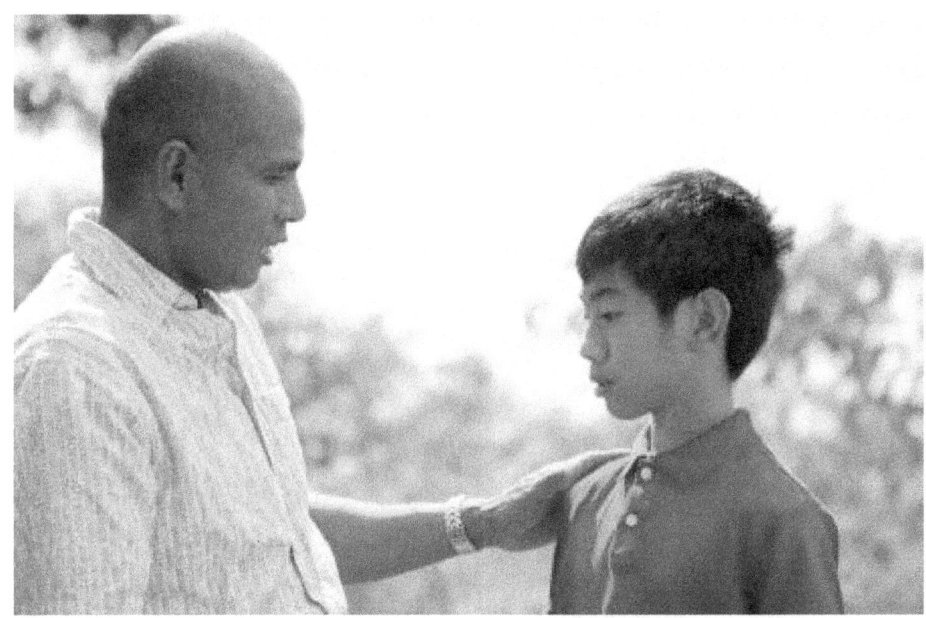

An autistic child cannot make friends, and that is why he/she going to suffer from loneliness, even though people are under the impression that they like to be alone. Nobody likes to be alone. That is why many of these children cannot express their helplessness when they are sidetracked from social events like invitations to picnics and parties.

Autistic children are going to respond abnormally to touch, towns, or other sensory stimulation. They may or may not be sensitive to pain. They can also display extraordinary sensitivity to other sensations. They made not like to be cuddled, or hugged.

This is the reason why many people, when confronted with autistic children get offended when the child shies away from any demonstration of affection. They do not know that it is possible that the child is sensitive to a touch, and maybe feeling pain when held physically.

Self-Injurious Behavior

Many children with autism are going to indulge in self injurious behavior. They may bang their heads or bite themselves. Just put yourself in that child's shoes. He understands what you are saying to him. You are going to be surprised to know that he understands more than you presume his supposed intellectual level is capable of comprehending.

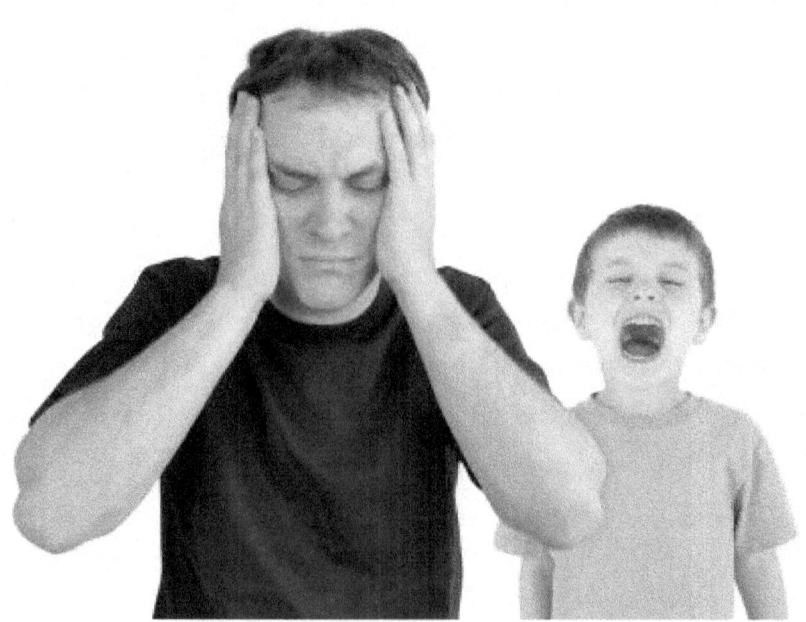

He wants to respond to you. But he cannot smile, put out a hand, laugh, and do all the other activities being done by children of his own age group. So that sort of helplessness is going to show, in some ways, a way he can gain attention.

This can only be done by screaming, or hurting himself physically. You respond immediately. In some corner of his mind, he understands that this sort of behavior is going to get attention, and get some sort of response from you. He is going to do this, whenever he wants attention, and that is why the idea that autistic children are violent, came into being.

Don't you think this explanation is a much more valid and reasonable answer for the supposed violent tendencies in autistic children, than those touted by researchers who immediately labeled children with autism to be more prone to violence?

A child suffering from Down's Syndrome is often very affectionate. But a child suffering from ASD is not going to be able to display that sort of emotional closeness with the members of the family.

That is the reason why normal people who are conditioned to accepted forms of social behavior keep away from these children, because ignorance about this particular disorder and its side effects prevents them from interacting with these children.

So when my friend's daughter cries when I come to visit her, I know she is showing that she is happy to see me, in her own particular way of communication. So I look at the ceiling and cry away to both our mutual satisfaction!

Recognition of Symptoms and Diagnosis

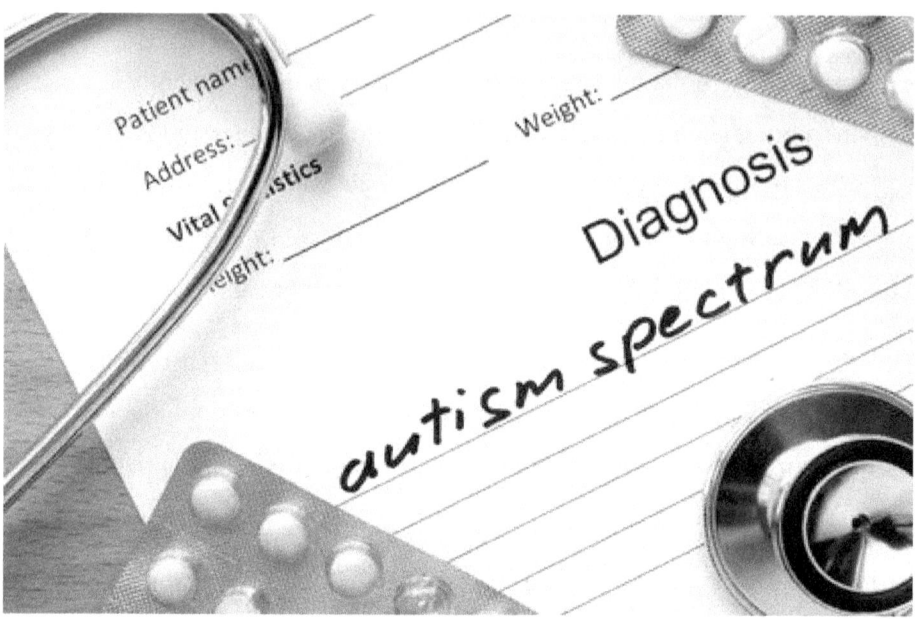

However, can these symptoms be recognized? It is possible for a parent to see certain symptoms as early as nine months. In nine months a normal child is normally going to point at things with his finger and babble some gibberish. By 16 months he is going to speak single words, and by 24 months. He is going to speak two word phrases. He is also going to communicate with you, verbally, especially when he wants something and right now!

Take these 3 age periods as your guide. If these things do not occur at these ages and the children show a lack of language or social skills at any age, they will need to be evaluated comprehensively.

The earlier you nab them, the better you will be able to treat them. Even at 18 months, you can recognize the fact that something is not well, a mother is going to notice some lack of reciprocity in the child. The child does not smile. The child also does not look at her mother and respond to any sort of verbal stimuli.

The speech is also not well developed. This child is also not going to ask for anything because it cannot communicate verbally. It may try to show its need for something through gestures.

For an 18 month child to be diagnosed as having a problem, the doctor or pediatrician should be aware of autism. He should also be able to recognize the symptoms on the basis of the observations related by the mother on the child's behavior and progress, or rather the lack of progress.

Diagnosis of Autism

There is absolutely no medical test with which you can diagnose autism doctors often describe an autistic person as being emotionally disturbed. This is their version of talking about a disorder about which they do not know much.

However, as autism symptoms vary differently depending on the cases and varying widely depending on the severity and the symptoms, many times autism is diagnosed strongly by doctors. They may even not recognize it, particularly in patients who are only mildly affected by it or who have other multiple disabilities.

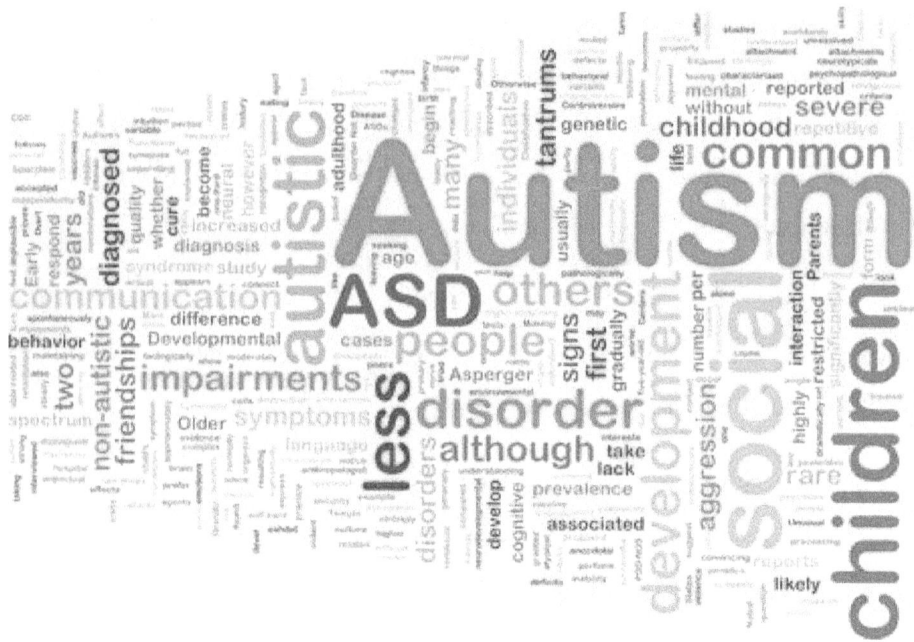

Usually, the medical fraternity based their diagnosis on certain features which are going to include –

1. Absence or lack of imaginative and social interaction.

2. Impaired ability to start or sustain a conversation with anybody.

3. Impaired ability to make friends with their own age group and peers and socialize with them.

4. Lack of spontaneous behavior, especially when one meets members of the family or while greeting acquaintances.

5. Stereotyped and repetitive behavior, actions, and language.

6. Restricted interests which are abnormally or intensely focused upon.

7. Preoccupation with some parts of objects and rigidity in following routines or rituals.

Is it possible for you to misdiagnose other conditions as autism, therefore making the diagnosis of autism that much more difficult? Well, doctors are not going to tell you that but there is a chance that doctors may listen to the symptoms and confuse them with some other disorder, or even symptoms that make up some other disorder, can be mistakenly diagnoses as autism!

For example, hearing impairment is also going to involve a delay in speech development. That is why a doctor might consider this to be possible autism, instead of treating the child for deafness.

And when the child has hearing problems coexisting with autism, the doctor is possibly justified in making sure he checks up the child's hearing before he reaches any conclusion and diagnoses the problem.

However, people suffering from Asperger's syndrome who also reveal autistic behavior are going to have well-developed language skills. Also, there are those children who appear normal in their earlier years. Then they start losing their skills and begin showing autistic behavior. These are the individuals with childhood disintegrative disorder.

Also, there are female children with Rett's syndrome, which is genetically influenced, here the girls manifest inadequate brain growth, have seizures, and other neurologic problems.

Savants are rare, but they are going to have extraordinary skills in music, mathematics, drawing, and visualization.

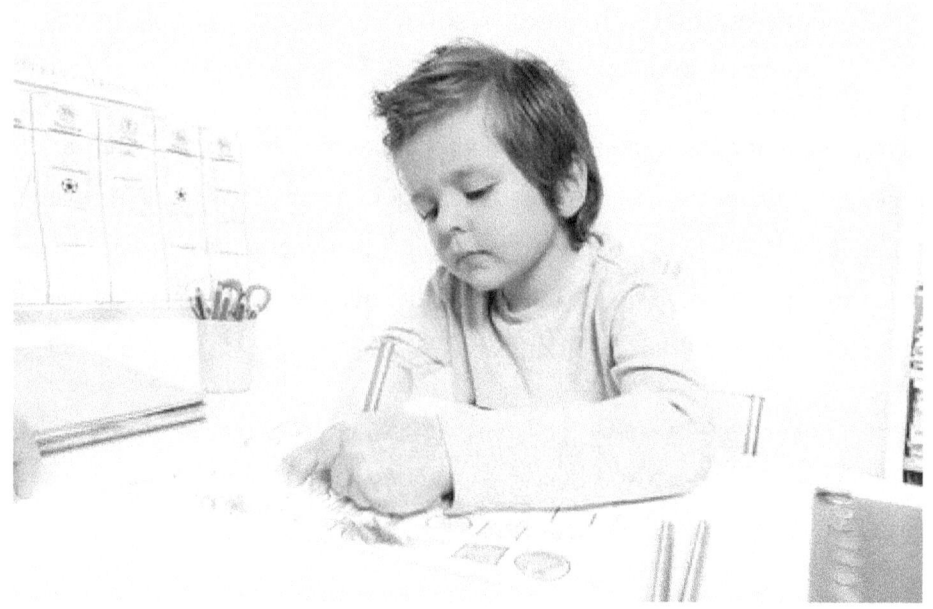

Treatment of Autism

It is a bit difficult to treat autism by medication. However, doctors talk about management of autism, rather than curing it. The medications are given to reduce or inhibit self-injurious behavior or even associated symptoms like epilepsy and attention disorders. However, their role in curing autism is rather limited.

There are a lot of alternative medicine treatments and nonmedicinal items like food products and vitamins which can to be given to a child. These are just supplements, but they are not the cure.

The most important aspect in treating autism is the management of the disorder through early intervention, and training.

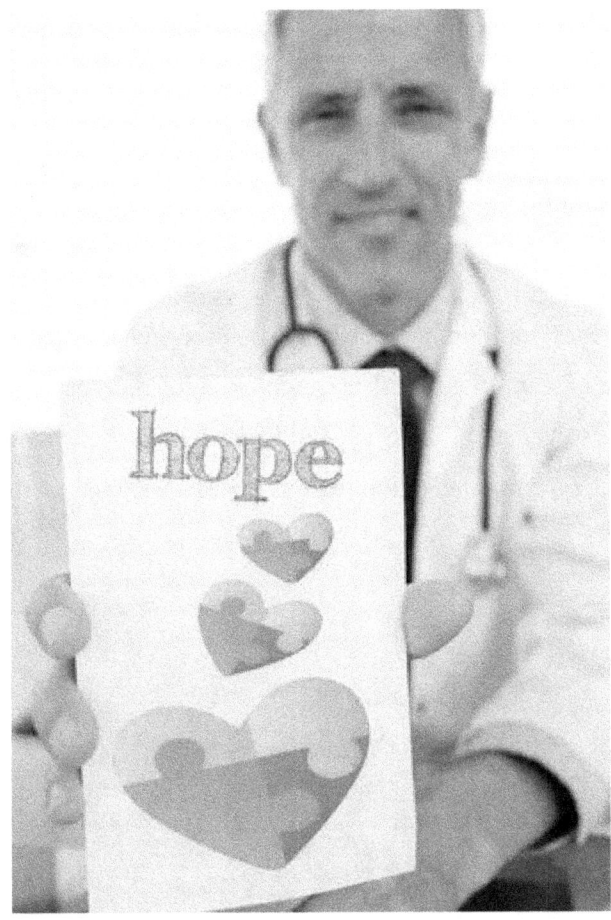

When the disorder is caught in its infancy and appropriate training techniques are adopted and reinforced persistently and consistently, there is going to be a reduction in the severity of emotional and behavioral upheavals in most instances.

These behavioral problems like violence and over activity occur often in autistic children, especially when they are nonverbal. As I told you before, here is this otherwise healthy little child, trying to communicate with you, but he cannot get his point across. How is he going to show his frustration and anger?

That is when he/she is going to do something violent and that is where early diagnosis and intuition, as well as, intervention is going to play an important role.

If the family does not train or teach the child properly and systematically the child is going to learn to get his/her way by kicking and resorting to other violent means to get attention. So as time goes by, he/she is going to consider it to be a communication pattern in order to "talk" to the adults around him/her.

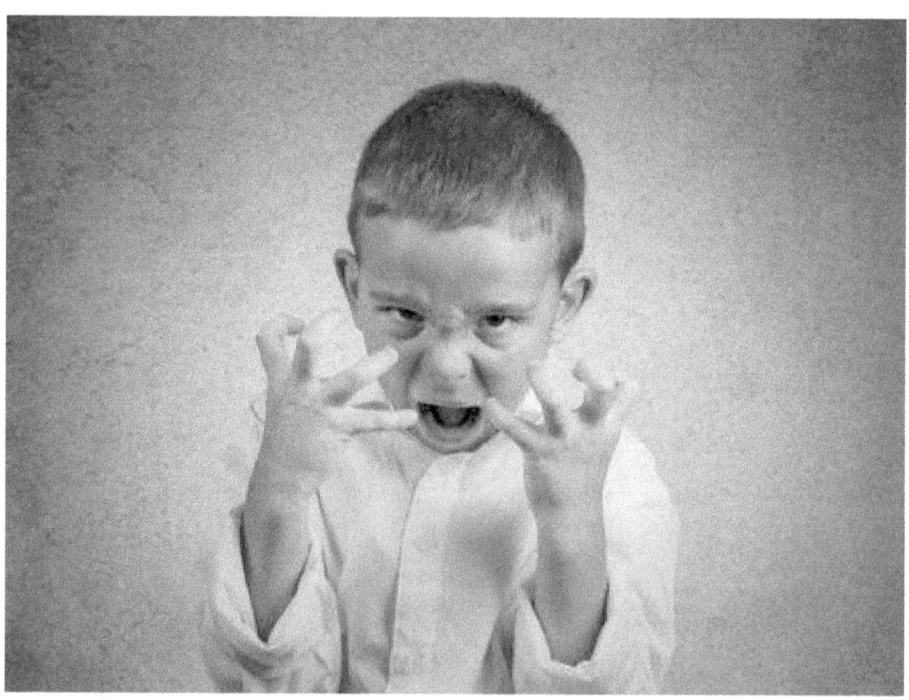

Such children have to be trained through visual communication with pictures. They can then understand how they can communicate and get their needs understood and fulfilled.

For example, if your child has a mild case of autism, and the family gives a lot of time in speech, and cognitive work, that child is going to be pushed to a state of normalcy. Yes, it can be done. The child may still have some odd and unusual behavior patterns, but one can hardly make them out.

A child who is very severely autistic with a great amount of training may come in the moderate category. One has heard of miracle cures, where autistic individuals have become normal. They are probably the people who have had an enormous and long-term amount of training.

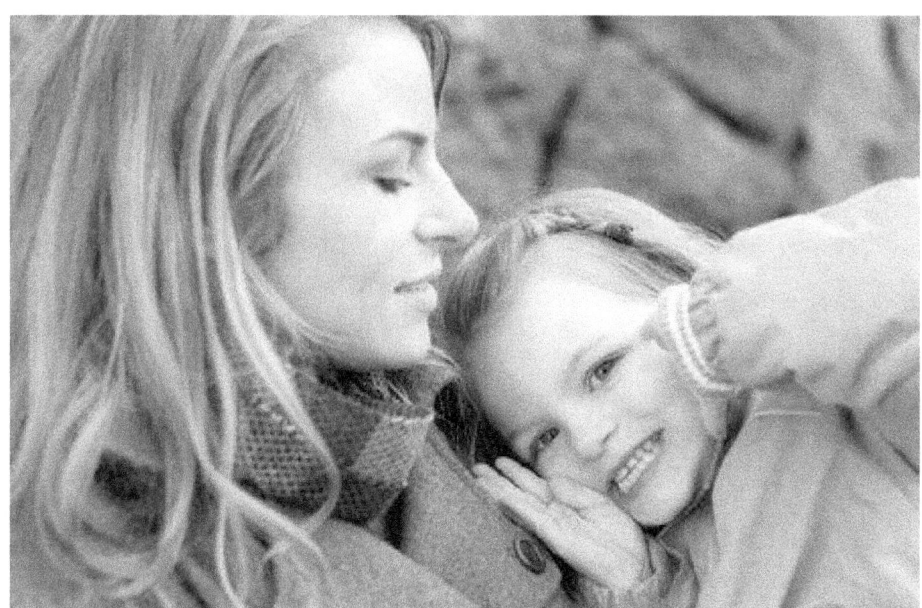

As signs of autism can be recognize as early as at 18 months, the mother of such a child will have embarked on immediate dedicated training. This is going to involve activities to stimulate speech, interact with the child in appropriate, enriching ways, with an 18 month old. Playing peek-a-boo, clapping hands, and playing such other games to draw him or her out of her shell and trying to establish a two-way communication process are some activities parents can do.

Hand stimulation, socialization and speech stimulation training will be good for any kind of development problem in which autism is one severe disorder.

Attitude of People towards Autistics

Like I told you before, there are many people out there who do not know much about autism. Believe it or not, 70% of these people consider these children to be mentally retarded. They club autism with mental retardation.

It is also true that many of these children may possibly be backward, but the word mental retardation is a psychological word which has been thought up by psychologists in order to explain something they considered abnormal or unusual.

Thanks to the Internet and forums on autism, more and more people are getting to know about this disorder. Especially when parents of such children are there to share their stories, and triumphs with other parents.

The reason why more and more people have become aware of autistic children being different from mentally retarded children is because the teaching and training methods for autism is very different in scope and content.

However, there are still places in many parts of the world where autism is considered to be a stigma, especially when the child is supposed to be abnormal or mad. Also, there are people who perceive the behavior of such children negatively, especially when they cannot understand why a child is not responding to their hello or does not want to be touched or hugged.

Also, believe it or not, there are plenty of medical specialists and doctors who still practice some beliefs which are consistent with research on thoroughly outmoded and outdated autism information. They are quite capable of telling you that your child is mentally retarded when he/she is just mildly autistic.

So here I come to the last and most important part of autism, the stress on the members of the family when there is an autistic child, demanding all the attention.

Stress on Family

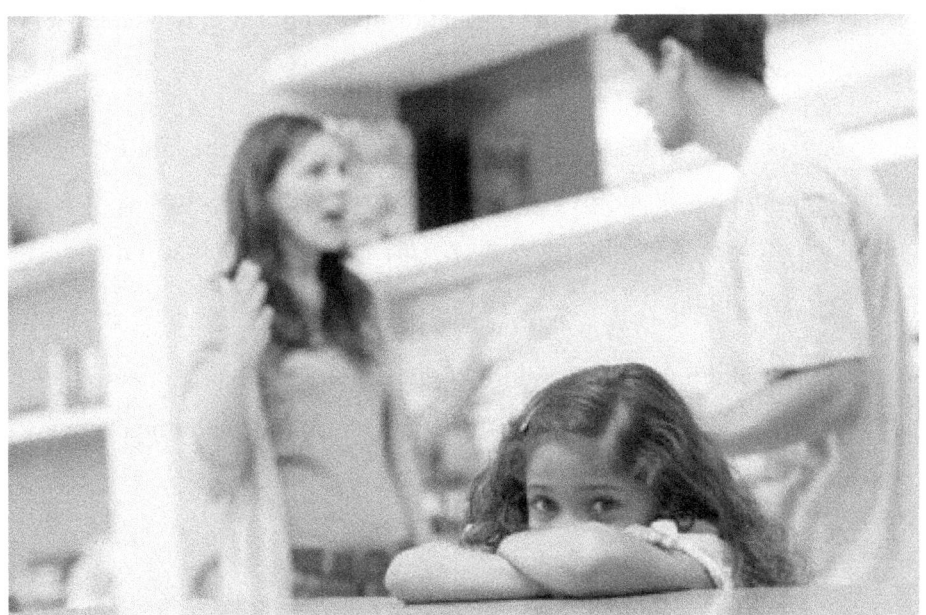

It is a well-researched fact that the stress on parents who have an autistic child is much more than stress and tension which parents of a normal child undergo. That is because the world still views autism as a social stigma. That is why they might find their social life to be restricted and circumscribed.

Thanks to online forums, such parents can continue being in touch with other parents in all the corners of the globe. Some of these parents consider autism to be a way of existence and accept it as a part of their lives. Others may keep looking for and hoping for a cure but with the support of other people, they managed to accept this part of their life.

Nevertheless, since a child suffering from autism takes up most of the mother's time and attention, the quality of her family life is going to suffer here. One is going to talk about the sibling attitude towards an autistic brother or sister. What is the kind of relationship with that may develop between them?

As an autistic child grows up, it becomes very attached to the family. It is going to do things with its siblings, though not activities that he has to do and which are normal for his or her age. That is because he is still in the process of learning.

A lot of these children have the ability to learn. So like all other neuro – developmental disorders, autism is also going to improve with the passage of time.

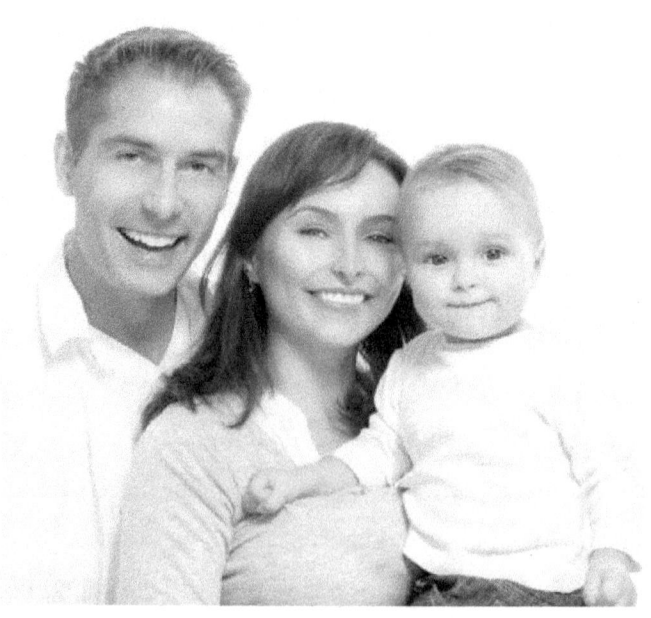

Some of the siblings of autistic children have behavioral problems because the autistic child takes up so much of the parents, particularly the mother's time, attention, and energy. Such marriages may also suffer, unless both partners are sensible and responsible enough to take on the upbringing of their child in a functional and practical manner. So instead of couples drifting apart because they are not aware and careful of what is happening to the quality of their own life together, they need to understand that the family is a solid unit.

It is undergoing a dynamic change. And everybody in the unit, including other children is going to contribute to the future happiness of the family and the quality of their life.

Conclusion

This book has given you plenty of information about autism, and how people with autistic children can still lead lives which are fulfilling, contented, and aware.

Remember, that discouragement is not an option. Giving your child lots of love, even if you cannot respond to you verbally is an option! Who knows, that he is sending you I love you messages telepathically? Your child may possibly become world famous one day, with lots of love and support from you. Even if he is not, after all, he is unique. They are your child.

I am giving you the example of Dr. Temple Grandin. She is autistic. She also did her doctorate in animal husbandry.

She built things that are necessary in large ranches to keep animals, including machinery, to soothe these animals. She remembered being hugged a lot by her mother when she was a baby, and this comforted her a lot, even though she could not express this verbally or emotionally.

She devised a machine which could be maneuvered in such a way as to bring the animals in their shed close together in a huddled fashion. Thus, they got plenty of comfort through physical contact with each other.

Live Long and Prosper!

Author Bio

Dueep Jyot Singh is a Management and IT Professional who managed to gather Postgraduate qualifications in Management and English and Degrees in Science, French and Education while pursuing different enjoyable career options like being an hospital administrator, IT,SEO and HRD Database Manager/ trainer, movie , radio and TV scriptwriter, theatre artiste and public speaker, lecturer in French, Marketing and Advertising, ex-Editor of Hearts On Fire (now known as Solstice) Books Missouri USA, advice columnist and cartoonist, publisher and Aviation School trainer, ex-moderator on Medico.in, banker, student councilor ,travelogue writer … among other things!

One fine morning, she decided that she had enough of killing herself by Degrees and went back to her first love -- writing. It's more enjoyable! She already has 48 published academic and 14 fiction- in- different- genre books under her belt.

When she is not designing websites or making Graphic design illustrations for clients , she is browsing through old bookshops hunting for treasures, of which she has an enviable collection – including R.L. Stevenson, O.Henry, Dornford Yates, Maurice Walsh, De Maupassant, Victor Hugo, Sapper, C.N. Williamson, "Bartimeus" and the crown of her collection- Dickens "The Old Curiosity Shop," and "Martin Chuzzlewit" and so on… Just call her "Renaissance Woman") - collecting herbal remedies, acting like Universal Helping Hand/Agony Aunt, or escaping to her dear mountains for a bit of exploring, collecting herbs and plants, and trekking.

Check out some of the other JD-Biz Publishing books

Gardening Series on Amazon

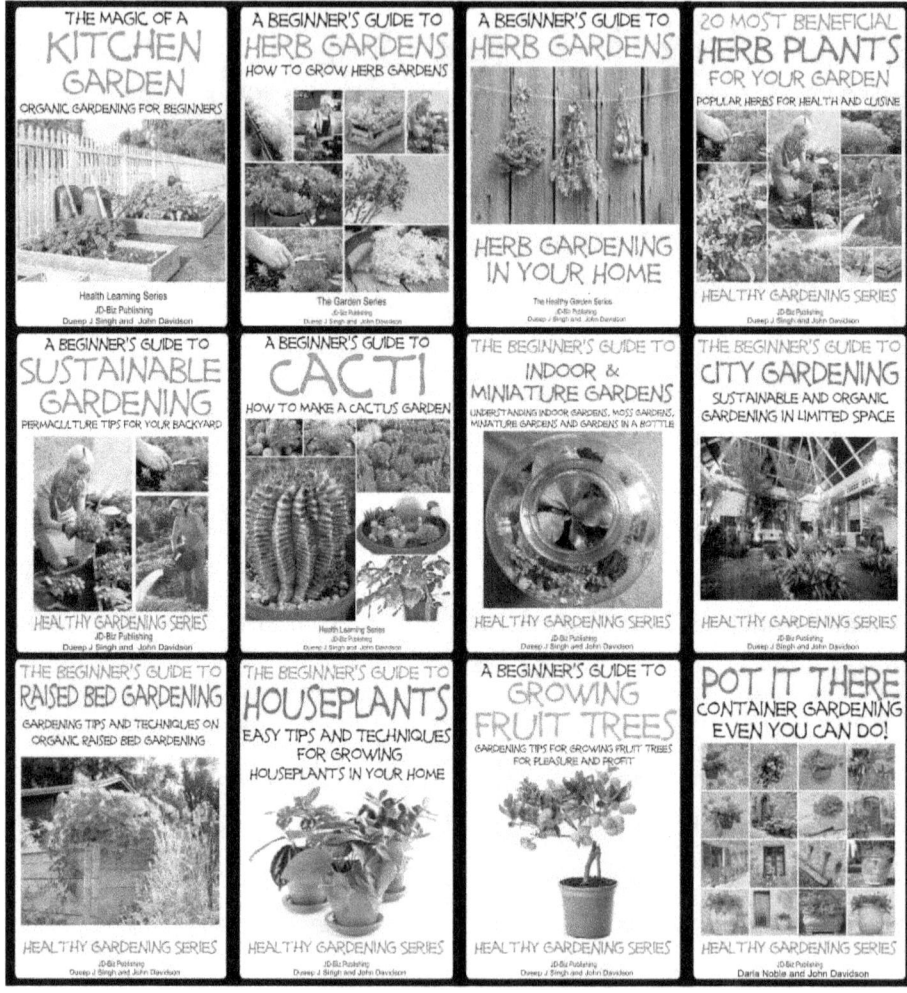

Health Learning Series

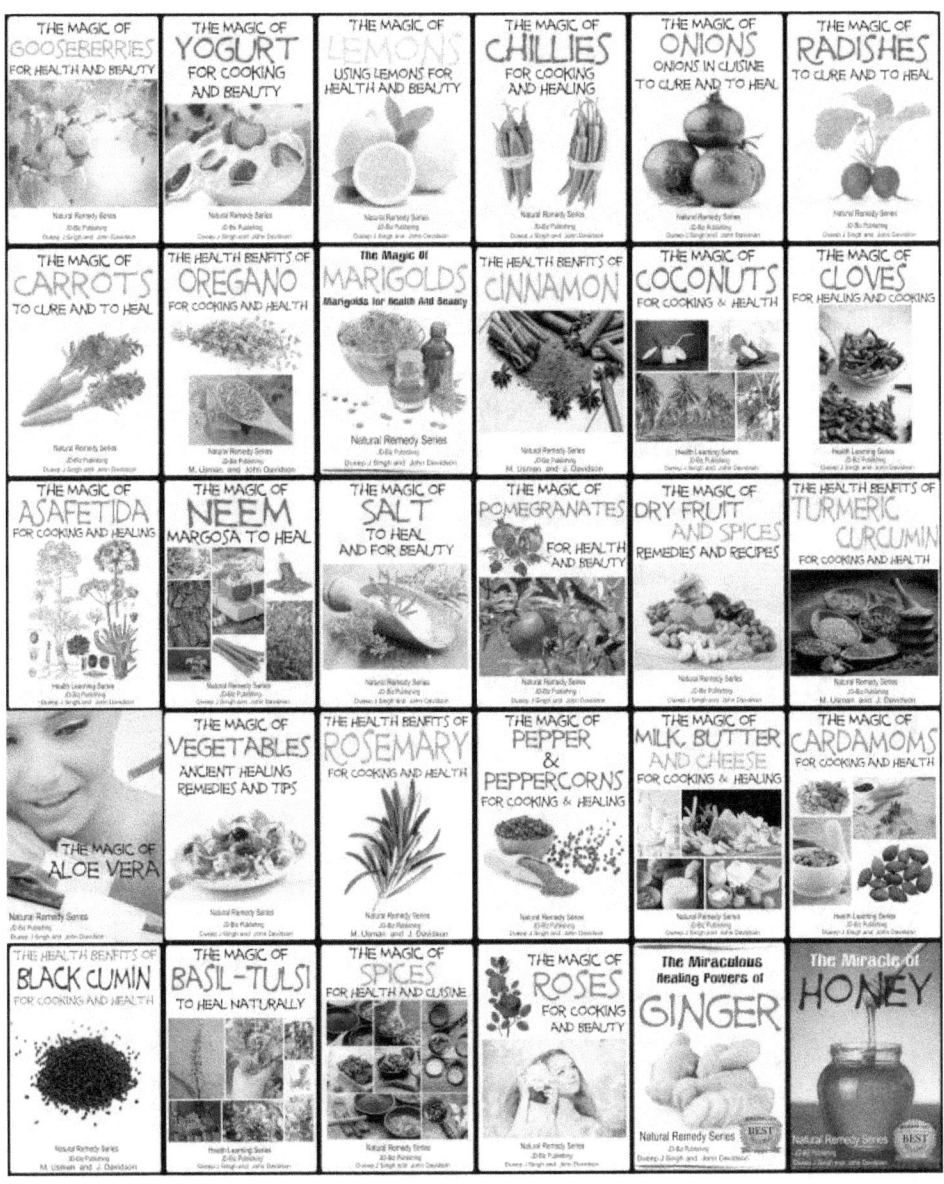

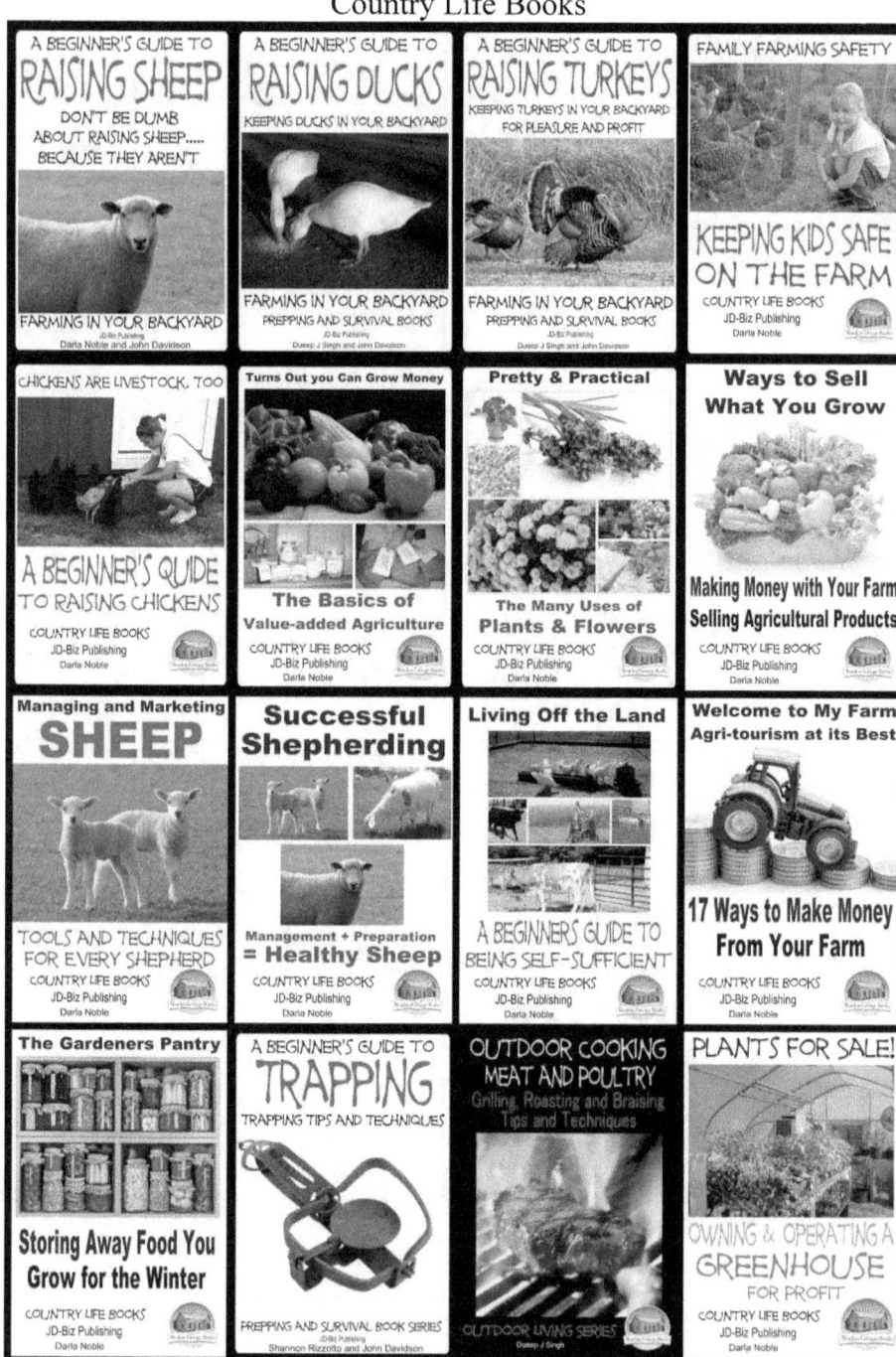

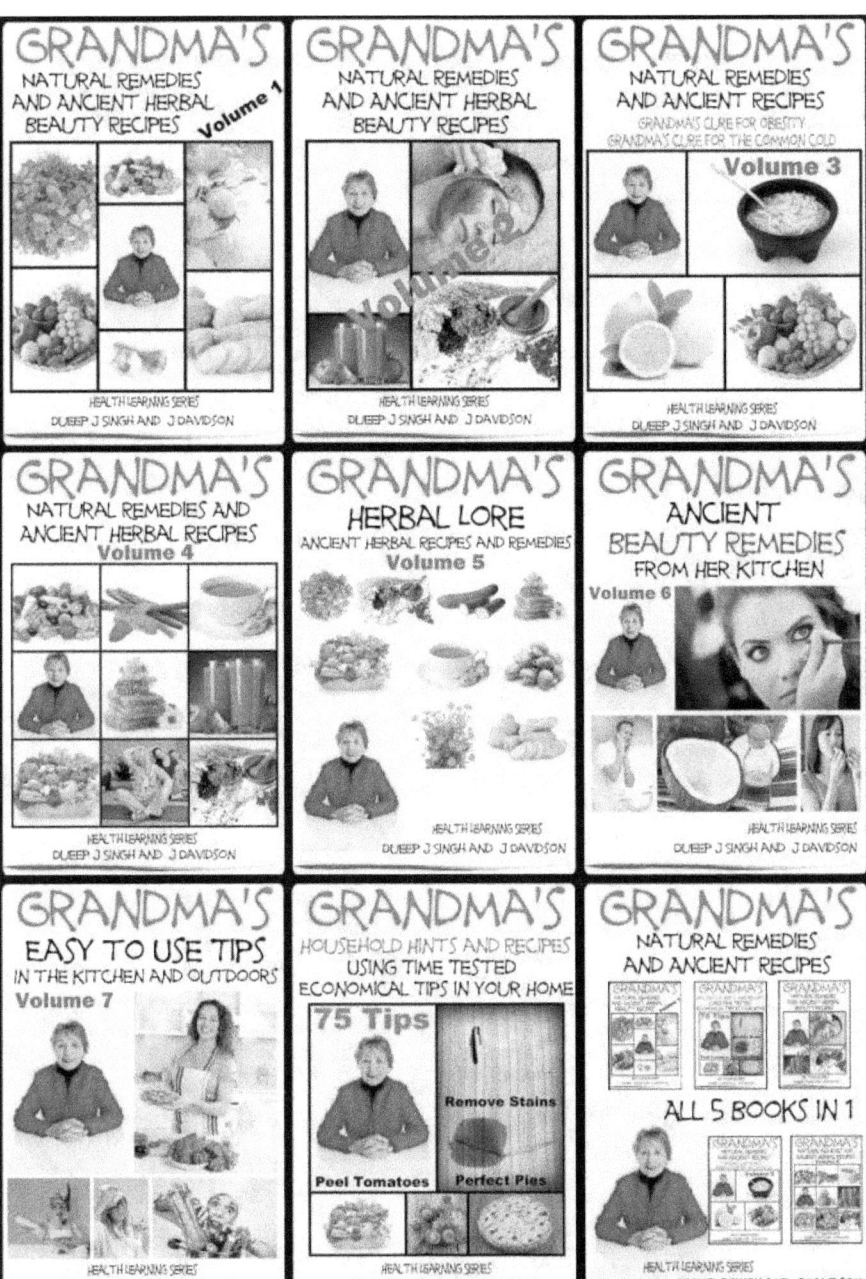

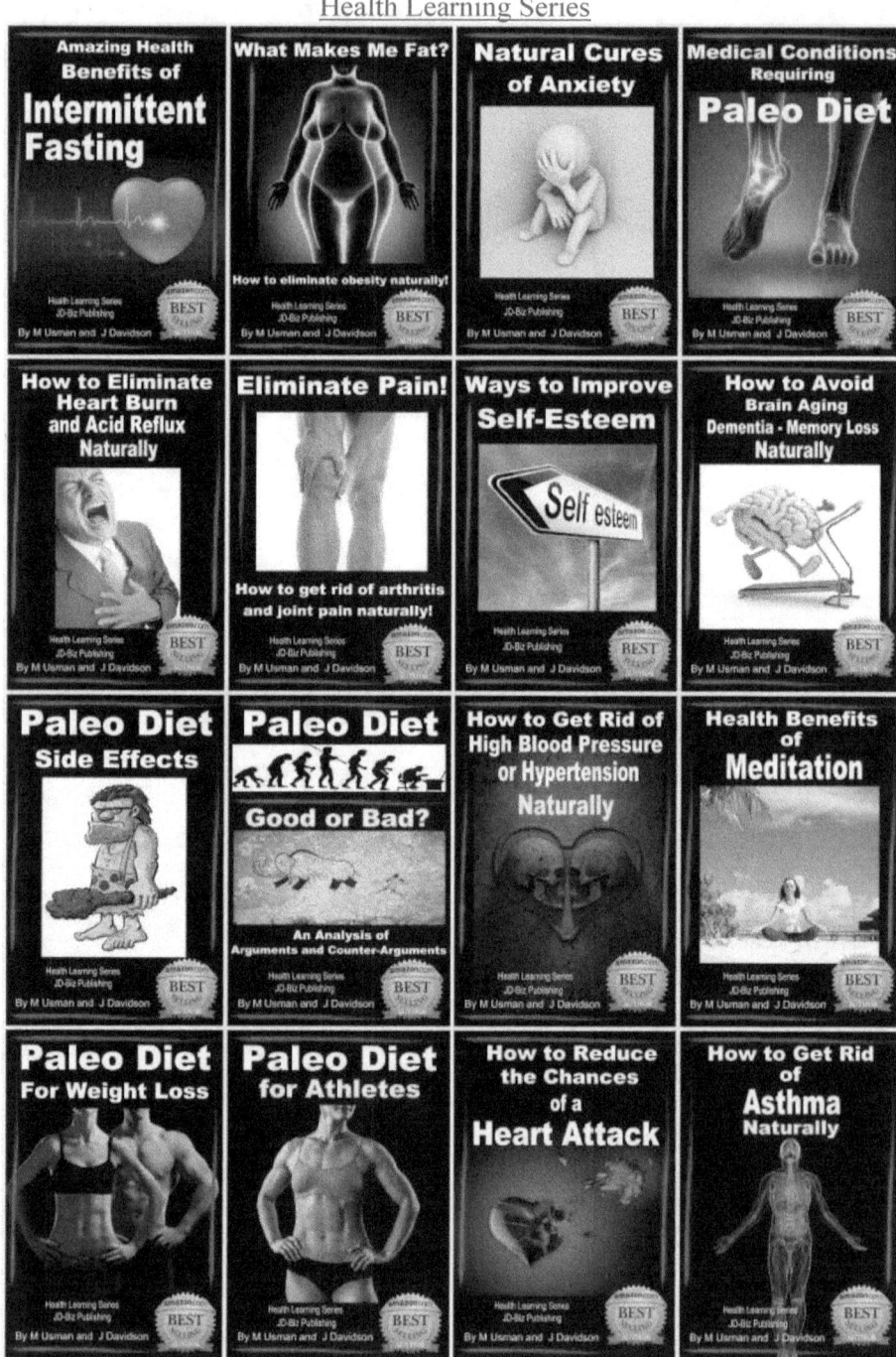

Amazing Animal Book Series

Learn To Draw Series

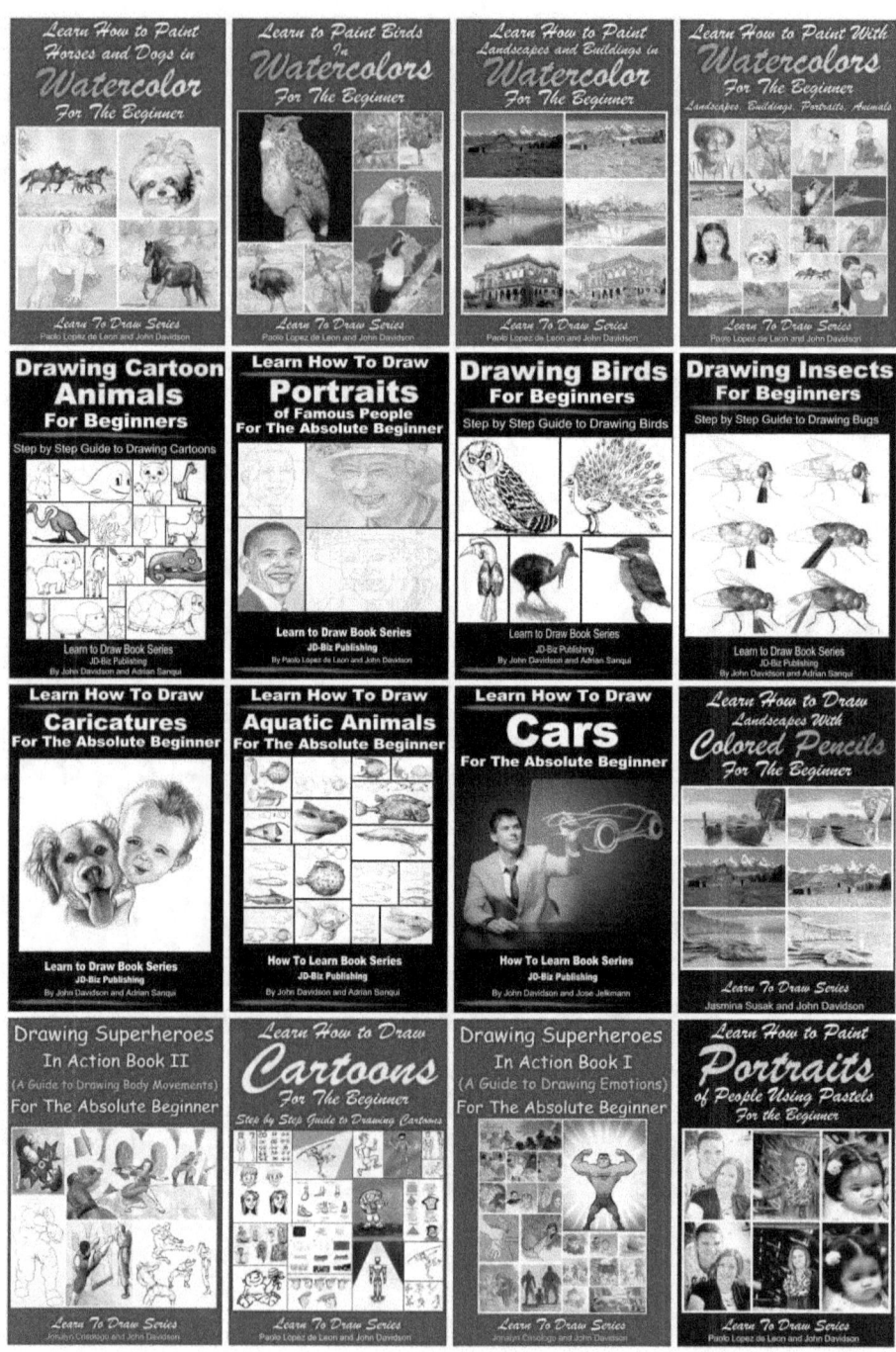

How to Build and Plan Books

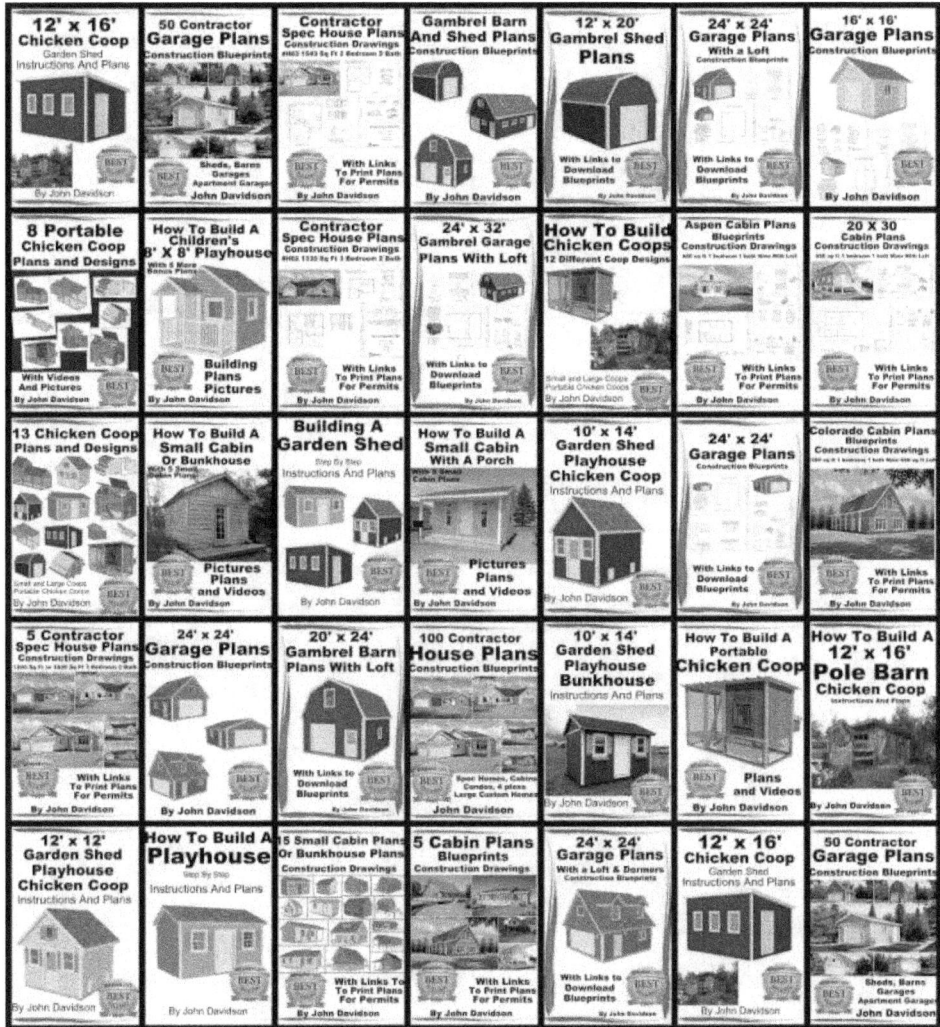

Entrepreneur Book Series

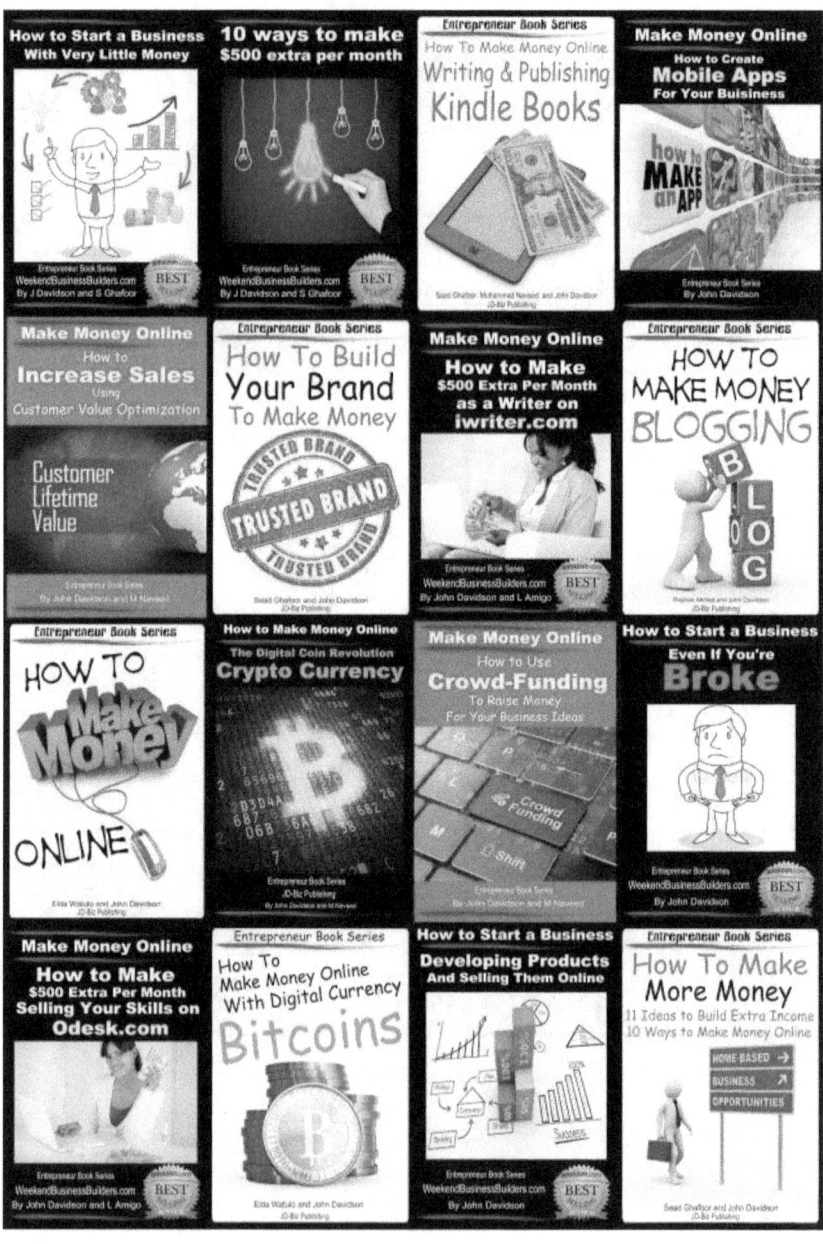

Our books are available at

1. Amazon.com

2. Barnes and Noble

3. Itunes

4. Kobo

5. Smashwords

6. Google Play Books

Publisher

JD-BIZ PUBLISHING

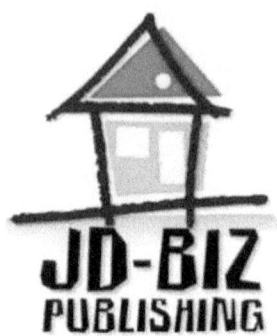

JD-Biz Corp

P O Box 374

Mendon, Utah 84325

http://www.jd-biz.com/

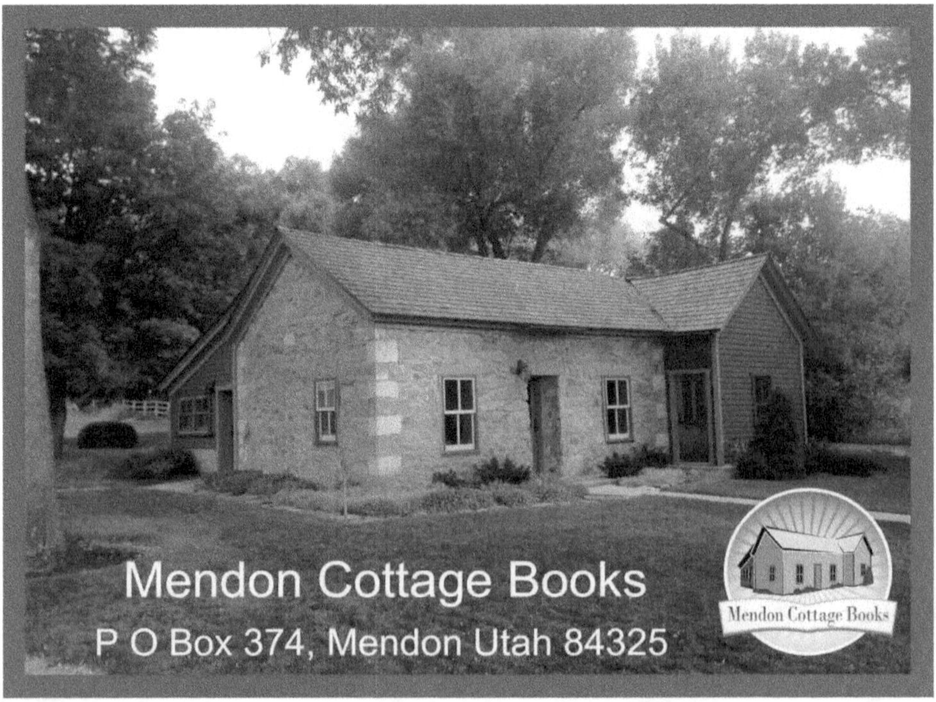

Mendon Cottage Books
P O Box 374, Mendon Utah 84325
Mendon Cottage Books

www.ingramcontent.com/pod-product-compliance
Lightning Source LLC
Chambersburg PA
CBHW070230210526
45168CB00019B/1351